[Year]

Myocardial infarction CAUSES-----

Cigarette smoking

Physical inactivity

a Fibrinogen

Hypertension

Obesity

a C-reactive protein   (this factor is uncertain)

Homocysteine

LDL cholesterol coronary disease Elevated Lp(a)

Low HDL

Increased cholesterol

Ethnicity

Diabetes mellitus

Psychosocial factors

Older age

Rx of CAD

disease with depressed LV function and left main stem coronary disease

Mitral Stenosis:

-causes of mitral stenosis are rheumatic fever,

Mid-diastolic murmur (best heard in expiration)

Loud S1, opening snap

Low volume pulse

Malar flush

Atrial fibrillation

Features of severe MS
Length of murmur
Opening snap becomes closer to S2

Echocardiography
The normal cross sectional area of the mitral valve is 4-6 cm2. A 'tight' mitral stenosis implies a cross sectional area of < 1 cm2.

Percutaneous Balloon Valvotomy: used to treat sever M.S.

Tricuspid Regurgitation:

Pan-systolic murmur

Giant v waves in JVP

Pulsatile hepatomegaly

Left parasternal heave

Causes of secondary hypertension

Renal m/c

Polycystic kidney disease

Chronic reflux nephropathy

Renal artery stenosis

Chronic glomerulonephritis

Polyarteritis nodosa

Conn's syndrome

Systemic sclerosis

Cushing's syndrome

Pheochromocytoma

Acromegaly

Hyperparathyroidism

Polycystic ovarian syndrome

diabetes mellitus,

dyslipidemia,

obesity

Pre-eclampsia

Obstructive sleep apnea

Aortic coarctation

combined oral contraceptive pill

, cyclosporin,

Steroid

raised intracranial pressure,

familial dysautonomia

Aortic dissection

Type A - ascending aorta - control BP(IV labetalol) + surgery

Type B - descending aorta - control BP(IV labetalol)

Primary Pulmonary Hypertension

Secondary causes of pulmonary hypertension include
COPD,

(Eisenmenger's syndrome)

Congenital heart disease

, recurrent pulmonary embolism,

HIV

and sarcoidosis.

Primary pulmonary hypertension
Pulmonary arterial pressure > 25 mmHg at rest, > 30mmHg with exercise

PPH is diagnosed when no underlying cause can be found

Around 10% of cases are familial: autosomal dominant

Endothelin thought to play a key role in pathogenesis

Associated with HIV,

cocaine

and anorexigens e.g. Fenfluramine

features
Cyanosis

Right ventricular heave

, loud P2,
raised JVP with prominent 'a' waves,

tricuspid regurgitation

rx
Diuretics if right heart failure

Anticoagulation

Vasodilator therapy:

calcium channel blocker,

IV prostaglandins, bosentan: endothelin-1
receptor antagonist

Heart-lung transplant

Pulmonary Arterial Hypertension (PAH) may be defined as a sustained elevation in
mean pulmonary arterial pressure of greater than 25 mmHg at rest or 30 mmHg after exercise.

Exertional dyspnea is the most frequent symptom

Chest pain and syncope may also occur

Loud P2

Left parasternal heave (due to right ventricular hypertrophy)

Idiopathic

Associated conditions: collagen vascular disease,

Familial

congenital heart disease with systemic to
pulmonary shunts,

HIV,

drugs and toxins,

sickle cell ds

HYPERTENSION Stage Signs

I   Arteriolar narrowing and tortuosity

Increased light reflex

"Silver wiring"

II Arteriovenous nipping

III Cotton-wool "exudates"

Flame and blot hemorrhages

IV Papilledema

Congenital heart disease

Cyanotic: TGA most common at birth,

Fallot's most common overall

Acyanotic: VSD most common cause

Tetralogy of Fallot is more common than transposition of the great arteries .

In newborn,
TGA is the most common presenting cause of cyanotic congenital heart disease.

Acyanotic - most common causes

Ventricular septal defects (VSD) - most common, accounts for 30%

Atrial septal defect (ASD)

Patent ductus arteriosus (PDA)

Coarctation of the aorta

Aortic valve stenosis

VSDs are more common than ASDs.

However, in adult patients ASDs are the more common new
diagnosis as they generally presents later

Cyanotic - most common causes

Tetralogy of Fallot

Transposition of the great arteries (TGA)
Tricuspid atresia

Pulmonary valve stenosis

Ventricular Septal defect

Atrial Septal Defects (ASDs)

adulthood. They carry a significant mortality, with 50% of patients being dead at 50 years

. Two types
of ASDs are recognised, ostium secundum and ostium primum.

Ostium secundum (70% of ASDs)

Associated with Holt-Oram syndrome

ECG: RBBB with RAD (secundum).

Ostium secundum are the most

splitting of S2

tri-phalangeal thumbs)

Coarctation of the Aorta

describes a congenital narrowing of the descending aorta

a/w

Infancy: heart failure

Adult: hypertension

Radio-femoral delay

Mid or late systolic murmur, maximal over back

Turner's syndrome

Bicuspid aortic valve

Berry aneurysms

Neurofibromatosis

Eisenmenger's Syndrome

is characterized by the reversal of the left-right shunt due to
pulmonary hypertention

a/w-
Cyanosis

Clubbing

Right ventricular failure

Hemoptysis,

Embolism

Rx-
Heart-lung transplantation is required

Tetralogy of Fallot (TOF)

is the most common cause of cyanotic congenital heart disease

It typically presents at around 1-2 months, although may not be picked up until the baby is 6
months
Old

The four characteristic features are:
Ventricular septal defect (VSD)

Right ventricular hypertrophy

Right ventricular outflow tract (RVOT) obstruction,

pulmonary stenosis

Overriding aorta

The severity of RVOT obstruction determines the degree of cyanosis and severity

Chest x-ray shows a 'boot-shaped' heart,

ECG shows right ventricular hypertrophy

hypertensive retinopathy Keith–Wagener classification

Resistant hypertension

Failure to reduce BP to <140/90 mm Hg with three or more drugs

ECG changes may be seen in hypothermia:

Bradycardia

'J' wave - small hump at the end of the QRS complex=osborn wave

First degree heart block

Long QT interval

J waves are seen in hypothermia

delta waves are associated with WPW

Jugular Venous Pulse:

A non-pulsatile JVP is seen in
superior vena caval obstruction.

Kussmaul's sign

describes a paradoxical rise in JVP during inspiration
seen in constrictive pericarditis.

Kussmaul's sign _ constrictive pericarditis

'a' wave = atrial contraction

Absent if in atrial fibrillation

Cannon 'a' waves

Are seen in complete heart block,

ventricular tachycardia/ectopics

single chamber ventricular pacing

Irregular cannon waves

Complete heart block

'c' wave

Closure of tricuspid valve

'v' wave

Giant v waves in tricuspid regurgitation

'x' descent Fall in atrial pressure during ventricular systole

'y' descent Opening of tricuspid valve

Heart Sounds:

The first heart sound (S1) is caused by closure of the mitral and tricuspid valves

the second heart sound (S2) is due to aortic and pulmonary valve closure

S1

Closure of mitral and tricuspid valves

Soft if long PR or mitral regurgitation

Loud in mitral stenosis

S2

closure of the aortic valve (A2) closely followed by that of the pulmonary valve (P2)

Causes of a loud S2

Hypertension: systemic (loud A2) or pulmonary (loud P2)

Hyperdynamic states

Causes of a soft S2

Aortic stenosis

fixed split S2

Atrial septal defect

Causes of a reversed (paradoxical) split S2 (P2 occurs before A2)

LBBB

Severe aortic stenosis

Right ventricular pacing

WPW type B

Patent ductus arteriosus

S3 •

Caused by diastolic filling of the ventricle

Considered normal if < 30 years old (may persist in women up to 50 years old)

Heard in left ventricular failure,

constrictive pericarditis

Gallop rhythm (S3) is an early sign of LVF

S4 •

heard in aortic stenosis,

HOCM,

Hypertension

caused by atrial contraction against a stiff ventricle

Pulses:

Pulsus parodoxus

Greater than the normal (10 mmHg) fall in systolic blood pressure during inspiration _ faint or absent pulse in inspiration

Severe asthma,

cardiac tamponade

Slow-rising/plateau——Aortic stenosis

Collapsing——

Aortic regurgitation

Patent ductus arteriosus

Hyperkinetic —

—(anemia, thyrotoxic, fever, exercise/pregnancy)

Pulsus alternans

Severe LVF

Bisferiens pulse

Mixed aortic valve disease

'Jerky' pulse

Hypertrophic obstructive cardiomyopathy

Causes of ST depression:

Ischemia

Digoxin

Hypokalemia

Syndrome X

Prolonged PR interval

PR interval is lengthened beyond 0.20 seconds (>5small squares)

Causes:
Idiopathic

Ischemic heart disease

Digoxin toxicity

Hypokalemia

Rheumatic fever

Lyme disease

Sarcoidosis

Myotonic dystrophy

Athletes

Hyperkalemia

Malignant (or accelerated phase) hypertension

In about 1% of patients with hypertension, BP is markedly raised (diastolic >130 mm Hg) and is associated with grade III–IV retinopathy.

CHF

The electrocardiogram of a patient with heart failure often shows LV hypertrophy (LVH).

Most commonly in the lateral chest leads.

Arrhythmias are also common in heart failure.

Chest x-ray

cardiomegaly

upper lobe blood diversion

"bat's wing" alveolar edema

pleural effusions

Kerley B lines (lymphatics) Management: acute heart failure

Acute pulmonary edema should be managed by:

Oxygen

diamorphine (intravenous [IV])

nitrates

loop diuretics

In left bundle branch block (LBBB), the pattern is best detected in V6 where there is an "M" pattern, while in V1 there is a "W"pattern

- In right bundle branch block (RBBB), the pattern is best detected in V1 where there is an RSR complex, while in V6 there is a QRS complex

Left anterior and left posterior fascicular block

Fascicular block causes axis deviation on the ECG. Therefore, left anterior hemiblock causes left axis deviation

left posterior hemiblock
causes right axis deviation

The term "bifascicular block" refers to a block of any two of the three fascicles.

- RBBB + left anterior hemiblock, ie, RBBB + left axis deviation

- RBBB + left posterior hemiblock, ie, RBBB + right axis deviation

Trifascicular block

Trifascicular block refers to a block of all three fascicles (but with intact AV conduction)

. It usually refers to LBBB + a long PR interval

Atrial tachycardia

rate varying from 140 to 240 bpm

Ventricular tachycardia

a very broad QRS complex (>0.14 seconds)

AV dissociation

fusion beats

capture beats

Atrial flutter

Atrial flutter is a rapid, regular rhythm with atrial rates of 250–350 bpm.

The ventricular response rate varies, but it is usually a 2:1 block

Aortic regurgitation

AR is associated with

waterhammer (collapsing) pulse

Corrigan's sign – visible arterial pulsation in the neck

de Musset's sign – nodding of the head in time with the heartbeat

Duroziez's sign – caused by retrograde diastolic flow in the femoral artery.

Quincke's sign – capillary pulsation in the nail beds that is visible

on applying gentle pressure to induce a degree of whitening
Traube's sign – a "pistol-shot" sound heard over the femoral pulse

Müller's sign – pulsation of the uvula

Rheumatic heart disease is the most common cause of MS

AF develops in 40% of patients with symptomatic MS

change from warfarin to heparin at week 36 in anticipation of labor

Duke diagnostic classification for IE

Cardiac temponade

A characteristic of cardiac tamponade is pulsus paradoxus, which is not paradoxical at all, but an exaggeration of the normal drop in systolic pressure on inspiration – >10 mm Hg is abnormal.

Low-voltage ECG and beat-to-beat variation in R-wave amplitude are characteristic.

CXRs show a globular, "boot-shaped" heart.

significant ascites

Constrictive pericarditis

raised JVP with positive Kussmaul

and Friedrich's signs

hepatomegaly

pulsus paradoxus (but usually less severe than in tamponade)

pericardial knock (high-pitched early diastolic added sound)

calcification visible on the lateral CXR

Primum ASD requires prophylaxis for infective endocarditis, while secundum ASD does not

RF

Major criteria for Rheumatic fever are: Chorea carditis polyarthritis erythema marginatum nodules (subcutaneous)
 Minor criteria are: fever arthralgia raised inflammatory markers previous rheumatic fever prolonged PR on ECG 2 major or 1 major and 2 minor satisfy criteria for Rheumatic Fever

Plus lab test of streptococci

Leads-

aVR lead: right arm

aVL lead: left arm

aVF lead: left leg

Axis Deviation-

Normal= -30 to +90

Ref-Many books

Left= -30 to -90

Right= +90 to +180

In Harrison --QRS axis ranges from -30° to +100° An axis more negative than -30° is called to as left axis deviation, while an axis more positive than +100° is called to as right axis deviation

MYOCARDIAL INFARCTION-ref.harrison

Acute coronary syndromes
occur when a thrombus forms at the site of rupture of an atherosclerotic
plaque and acutely occludes a coronary artery

Levine's sign-
In acute myocardial infarction the patient often describes the pain by clenching fist

ECG

. The earliest changes are tall, positive, hyperacute T waves .
followed by elevation of the ST segments due to myocardial "injury pattern"
Over hours to days, T-wave inversion occurs
Lastly diminished R-wave amplitude or Q waves occur

ECG can indicate the location of the ischemia or infarction:
Anterior -leads V2 through V4
lateral –leads I, aVL,V5, and V6
inferior leads– II, III, aVF
posterior –R waves in leads V1 and V2.

Markers-
 serum myoglobin or CK-MB
Troponin T is also useful because it has a large diagnostic window, as it is increased from 12
hours to 10 days after myocardial infarction

t/t- oxygen and
nitroglycerin,.then Aspirin
acute STEMI present within 2 to 3 hours of symptom
onset then do PCI ideally within 90 minutes
 anticoagulation -heparin and glycoprotein IIB/IIIA
 beta-blockers are used to decrease
myocardial oxygen demand,
nitrates are given
streptokinase,alteplase

TIMI grades-
 the Thrombolysis in Myocardial Infarction trial (TIMI) that measure coronary blood
flow & luminal narrowing:
· Grade 0: no flow of contrast beyond the point of occlusion.
· Grade I: penetration with minimal perfusion
· Grade 2: partial perfusion
· Grade 3: Complete perfusion
Evaluation of LV systolic function

Bypass surgery may be indicated for
patients with multivessel stenosis and impaired systolic function to reduce
symptoms and prolong survival.

complication -Life-threatening ventricular arrhythmias, such as ventricular tachycardia
(VT) and ventricular fibrillation (VF), are common—treat with direct current (DC) cardioversion,
followed by infusion
and intravenous antiarrhythmics such as amiodarone

Sinus bradycardia is   frequently seen in inferior MI
Cardiogenic shock is diagnosed
when the patient has hypotension with systolic arterial pressure less
than 80 mm Hg, markedly reduced cardiac index less than 1.8 L/min/m2, and
elevated capillary wedge pressure>18 mm HG
 Hypotension may also be seen in patients with right ventricular (RV) infarction
RV function is
impaired ,treat by
 volume replacement with saline or colloid solution

complication m/c-most common is papillary muscle dysfunction
Late complications that occur several weeks after an acute MI include development
of a ventricular aneurysm, which should be suspected if ST-segment elevation
persists weeks after the event

 Dressler syndrome, an immune
phenomenon characterized by pericarditis, pleuritis, and fever. Dressler syndrome
may remit and relapse, and it is treated with anti-inflammatory drugs and sometimes steroids

Post-MI patients with severe LV
dysfunction (LV ejection fraction

<30%-35%) are at increased risk for sudden
cardiac death from ventricular arrhythmias

First-degree AV block (PR-interval prolongation)
 Mobitz I seconddegree–AV block (gradual prolongation of the PR interval)
 Mobitz II second-degree AV block –nonconducted P
waves not preceded by PR prolongation
third-degree AV block ––complete
AV dissociation with no P-wave conduction

Causes of left axis deviation -

Ref-harrison

Left anterior hemiblock

Left bundle branch block

Hyperkalemia

Wolff-parkinson-white syndrome- rightsided
accessory pathway

Congenital: ostium primum ASD,

tricuspid atresia

Cause of right axis deviation

Ref-harrison

Right ventricular hypertrophy

Chronic lung disease

Left posterior hemiblock

Pulmonary embolism

Ostium secundum ASD

Wolff-parkinson-white syndrome – leftsided accessory pathway

Association---

Ref-harrison

Marfan's syndrome— Aortic regurgitation (aortic dissection)

Down's syndrome —ASD, VSD

Turner's syndrome —Coarctation of the aorta

Ankylosing spondylitis — Aortic regurgitation

First-degree AV block

This is where there is a prolonged PR interval of >200 milliseconds
No specific therapy is required and the prognosis is excellent.

Second-degree AV block

two types:
- type I (Mobitz I or Wenckebach AV block)
- type II (Mobitz II AV block)

Type I occurs when there is a repeated pattern of progressive prolongation of the
PR interval, which eventually results in the failure of conduction of one atrial beat
T Routine prophylactic permanent pacing is not recommended unless
the patient is symptomatic

type II— constant PR interval, but occasionally
atrial depolarization is not followed by ventricular depolarization .

Type II is pathological and It can lead to complete AV block, causing Stokes–Adams attacks. So, temporary and then permanent pacing is indicated in most patients, even those who initially present without symptoms.

Third-degree AV block (complete heart block)

there is complete dissociation of the P waves and QRS complexes

There is a significant risk of asystole and thus permanent pacing is indicated

Pericarditis:

Causes

Viral infections (Coxsackie)

Uremia (causes 'fibrinous' pericarditis)

TB

Trauma

Post MI, Dressler's syndrome

Connective tissue diseases

Hypothyroidism

ECG changes.
Widespread 'saddle-shaped' ST elevation

a/w

Clubbing —— Infective endocarditis,

ROTH SPOTS: Hemorrhagic retinal lesions with white center – infectious endocarditis

Splinter Streak hemorrorage—Infective endocarditis

Janeway lesions — Infective endocarditis

Osler's nodes Tender nodules — Infective endocarditis

Hypertension

PREHYPERTENSION: Blood pressures 120 to 139/80 to 89 mm Hg

STAGE I HYPERTENSION: Blood pressures 140 to 159/90 to 99 mm Hg

STAGE II HYPERTENSION: Blood pressures more than 160/100 mm Hg

Aim of t/t
target blood pressure is 135/85 mm Hg,
in pt with diabetes or renal disease   target would be lower than 130/80 mm Hg.

Most common cause of endocarditis:

Streptococcus viridans

Staphylococcus epidermidis if < 2 months post valve surgery

large majority of rightsided endocarditis is caused by Staphylococcus aureus.

m/c investigation for IE=TEE transesophageal echocardiography

DUKE CRITERIA FOR DIAGNOSIS OF ENDOCARDITIS
Major criteria
Isolation of typical organisms from two separate blood cultures
Evidence of endocardial involvement

Minor criteria
Fever 38 C or 100.4F
•Predisposing valvular lesion or intravenous drug use

Vascular phenomena: arterial or septic pulmonary emboli,janeway lesion , mycotic aneurysm
immunologic phenomena: posive rheumatoid factor, glomerulonephritis, Osler nodes, Roth
spot

Positive blood cultures not meeting major criteria

Cardiac Tamponade:

Raised JVP, with an absent Y descent - this is due to the limited right ventricular filling

Tachycardia

Hypotension

Muffled heart sounds

Pulsus paradoxus (which occurs also in Asthma)

Kussmaul's sign — (more in constrictive pericarditis)

Cardiac tamponade requires urgent treatment by pericardiocentesis or a pericardial window

Acute pericarditis=pleural rub ,fever and elevated T wave

Match box

Malar flush Redness around the cheeks— Mitral stenosis

Xanthomata Yellowish deposit in the Hyperlipidemic

Corneal arcus A ring around the cornea –in old Age, hyperlipidemia

Myocardial Infarction (MI):

Coronary Circulation (arterial supply of the heart)

Posterior aortic or coronary sinus _ left coronary artery (LCA)

Anterior aortic or coronary sinus _ right coronary artery (RCA)

LCA (Left Main, LM) _ LAD + circumflexRCA _ posterior descending

RCA supplies SA node in 60%, AV node in 90%

Venous drainage of the heart: coronary sinus drains into the right atrium

Anteroseptal V1-V4 Left anterior descending

Inferior II, III, aVF Right coronary

Anterolateral V4-6, I, aVL Left anterior descending or left circumflex

Lateral I, aVL +/- V5-6 Left circumflex

Posterior Tall R waves V1-2 Usually left circumflex

Rx-
ACE inhibitor
-blocker
Aspirin
Statin

RHEUMATIC HEART DISEASE

mitral valve is most frequently involved

Pulse---

Regularly irregular – 2nd-degree heart block,

Irregularly irregular – Atrial fibrillation,

Slow rising Low gradient upstroke-- Aortic stenosis

Water hammer----Aortic regurgitation,

Bisferiens A double-peaked pulse – the Aortic regurgitationhypertrophic cardiomyopathy

Pulsus paradoxus An exaggerated fall in pulse Cardiac tamponade,

Bounding Large volume pulse--Anemia, hepatic failure,
type 2 respiratory failure
(high CO2)

Causes of long QT interval

Congenital: Jervell-Lange-Nielsen syndrome, Romano-Ward syndrome

Antiarrhythmics: amiodarone, sotalol, class I-a antiarrhythmic drugs

Tricyclic antidepressants

Antipsychotics

Chloroquine

quinidine,

disopyramide,

procainamide,

Terfenadine

Erythromycin

Hypocalcemia,

Hypokalemia,

Hypomagnesemia

Myocarditis

Hypothermia

Subarachnoid haemorrhage

Amiodarone

Sotalol

Romano–Ward syndrome

Flecainide

Pulmonary embolism

Sinus tachycardia is seen in pulmonary embolism. New right
bundle branch block (RBBB) or right axis deviation with "strain" can also indicate
PE. The classic SIQIIITIII is less common

Hyperkalemia

tall, tented T waves

lengthening of the PR interval

reduction in the P-wave height

widening of the QRS complex

"sinus" wave QRS pattern

Hypokalemia

Flat T wave

U WAVE

ST DEPRESSION

PROLONG PR

Long QT Syndrome (LQTS)

is an inherited condition, The most common variants of LQTS (LQT1 & LQT2) are caused by defects in slow delayed rectifier potassium channel.

A normal corrected
QT is less than 440 ms in _s and 450 ms in _s.

Blockage of K+ channels causes prolongation of QT

Rx of hypekalemia

A sinus-wave QRS should be treated immediately with calcium chloride

hyperkalemia associated with lesser ECG changes can be treated with insulin/glucose infusion

SEVERE HYPERKALEMIA

ASYSTOLE

WIDE QRS

SINE WAVE

VENTRICULAR TACHYCARDIA

VENTRICULAR FIBRILLATION

The JVP should be assessed with the patient reclined at a 45° angle

Wolff-Parkinson White (WPW)

syndrome is caused by a congenital accessory conducting
pathway between the atria and ventricles leading to atrioventricular re-entry tachycardia (AVRT).

As
the accessory pathway does not slow conduction AF can degenerate rapidly to VF

Possible ECG features include:

Short PR interval

Wide QRS complexes with a slurred upstroke - 'delta wave'

Left axis deviation if right-sided accessory pathway

Right axis deviation if left-sided accessory pathway

Steep "x", "y" descent— Constrictive pericarditis, cardiac tamponade

Large "v" wave, "cv" wave —Tricuspid regurgitation

Kussmaul's sign— Rise of JVP on inspiration, constrictive pericarditis, cardiac tamponade

Large "a" wave —Tricuspid stenosis, pulmonary hypertension, pulmonary stenosis

ı

Cannon wave ——Atrial fibrillation, complete heart block,

Brugada syndrome –

. It is inherited in an autosomal dominant fashion and has an estimated prevalence of 1:5,000-10,000.

Brugada syndrome is more common in Asians.

A large number of variants exist

Around 20-40% of cases are caused by a mutation in the SCN5a gene which encodes the myocardial sodium ion channel protein

Convex ST elevation V1-V3

Partial right bundle branch block

Changes may be more apparent following Flecainide

Brugada pattern —right bundle branch block-like pattern with ST elevations in right precordial leads

(class la antiarrhythmic) is used to
unmaks hidden Brugada

Patients do not benefit from beta blocker therapy. Sodium channel-blocking drugs, such as
procainamide and flecainide, can exacerbate the syndrome
Implantable cardioverter-defibrillator done

Quinidine is useful in VF

Transesophageal echocardiography

The key indications for TEE are:

infective endocarditis – if vegetations are not seen on transthoracic echo,
but suspicion is high, or with prosthetic valves
to rule out an embolic source (especially in atrial fibrillation)

acute dissection

mitral valve (MV) disease preoperatively

lead	
Inferior II, III, aVF	
Anterior I, aVL, V1–V3	
Septal V3, V4	
Lateral V4–V6	

small Q waves correspond to depolarization of the interventricular septum. They can signal an old myocardial infarction (in which case they are big and wide)

- the R wave reflects depolarization of the main mass of the ventricles – hence it is the largest wave

- the S wave signifies the final depolarization of the ventricles

T waves represent ventricular repolarization (atrial repolarization is obscured by the large QRS complex).

Hypertrophic Obstructive Cardiomyopathy (HOCM)

is an autosomal dominant

disorder of muscle tissue caused by defects in the genes encoding contractile proteins.

The estimated prevalence is 1 in 500.

Septal hypertrophy causes left ventricular outflow obstruction. It is an important cause of sudden death in apparently healthy individuals.

Hypertrophic obstructive cardiomyopathy (HOCM) is a more common cause of sudden cardiac death than arrhythmogenic right ventricular dysplasia (ARVD) _ 2nd most common

Often asymptomatic

Dyspnea, angina, syncope

Sudden death (most commonly due to ventricular arrhythmias), arrhythmias, heart failure

Jerky pulse,

large 'a' waves

, double apex beat

Ejection systolic murmur: _ with valsalva manoeuvre and _ on squatting

a/w

Friedreich's ataxia

Wolff-Parkinson White syndrome

Left ventricular hypertrophy (LVH)

Atrial enlargement (abnormal P morphology)

Progressive T wave inversion

ST-T abnormalities

Deep Q waves

Axis deviation

Prolonged PR or sinus bradycardia

BBB (bundle brach block)

No P waves and irregular narrow QRS complexes This is hallmark of atrial fibrillation

Sawtooth P waves
A sawtooth waveform signifies atrial flutter

Long PR interval
sign of hyperkalemia, digoxin toxicity, or cardiomyopathy

A wide QRS complex despite sinus rhythm is the hallmark of bundle branch block

Hypertrophic cardiomyopathy

echo remains the screening tool of choice in suspected cases. The classic features are asymmetrical hypertrophy of the interventricular septum and anterior movement of the MV in systole . LV function

is normal, and there may be dynamic LV outflow tract obstruction.

pulsus parvus, is common in conditions with a diminished left ventricular stroke volume

pulsus tardus, results from obstruction to left ventricular ejection

Pulsus alternans—LVF

c wave, often observed in the JVP is a positive wave produced by the bulging of the tricuspid valve into the right atrium during right ventricular isovolumetric systole and by the impact of the carotid artery adjacent to the jugular vein

The x descent is due both to atrial relaxation and to the downward displacement of the tricuspid valve during ventricular systole.

y descent of the JVP—is produced mainly by the opening of the tricuspid valve and the subsequent rapid inflow of blood into the right ventricle. A rapid, deep y descent in early diastole occurs with severe tricuspid regurgitation v wave results from the increasing volume of blood in the right atrium during ventricular systole when the tricuspid valve is closed

Large a waves indicate that the right atrium is contracting against an increased resistance, such as occurs with tricuspid stenosis or more commonly with increased resistance to right ventricular filling pulmonary hypertension or pulmonic stenosis

a wave is absent in patients with atrial fibrillation

reverse splitting -Splitting is maximal in expiration and decreases during inspiration with the normal delay of pulmonic valve closure. The most common causes of reversed splitting of S_2 are left bundle branch block and delayed excitation of the left ventricle from a right ventricular ectopic beat

s4—systemic hypertension, aortic stenosis, hypertrophic cardiomyopathy, ischemic heart disease, and acute mitral regurgitation

S_3 usually indicates impairment of ventricular function, AV valve regurgitation

Holosystolic murmurs a/w mitral or tricuspid regurgitation and ventricular septal defect.

Continuous murmurs may result from congenital or acquired systemic arteriovenous fistula, coronary arteriovenous fistula, anomalous origin of the left coronary artery from the pulmonary artery, and communications between the sinus of Valsalva and the right side of the heart

The QRS complex represents ventricular depolarization, and the ST-T-U complex (ST segment, T wave, and U wave) represents ventricular repolarization. The J point is the junction between the end of the QRS complex and the beginning of the ST segment

ECG paper speed is generally 25 mm/s, the smallest (1 mm) horizontal divisions correspond to 0.04 (40 ms), with heavier lines at intervals of 0.20 s (200 ms

Vertically, the ECG graph measures the amplitude of a given wave or deflection (1 mV = 10 mm with standard calibration

lead I = left arm – right arm voltages, lead II = left leg – right arm, and lead III = left leg – left arm

normal atrial depolarization vector is oriented downward and toward the subject's left

QRS axis ranges from –30° to +100° An axis more negative than –30° is referred to as left axis deviation, while an axis more positive than +100° is referred to as right axis deviation---harrison

U-wave amplitude is most commonly due to drugs (e.g., dofetilide, amiodarone, sotalol, quinidine, procainamide, disopyramide) or to hypokalemia

Right ventricular hypertrophy due to a pressure load (as from pulmonic valve stenosis or pulmonary artery hypertension) is characterized by a relatively tall R wave in lead V_1 (R S wave), usually with right axis deviation alternatively, there may be a qR pattern in V_1 or V_3R

pulmonary embolism ---- Sinus tachycardia is the most common arrhythmia

coronary vasospasm (Prinzmetal's variant angina, and possibly the tako-tsubo cardiomyopathy syndrome), may cause transient ST-segment elevations without development of Q waves

Brugada pattern right bundle branch block-like pattern with ST elevations in right precordial leads

Hyperkalemia produces peaking (tenting) of the T waves. Further elevation of extracellular K^+ leads to AV conduction disturbances, diminution in P-wave amplitude, and widening of the QRS interval. Severe hyperkalemia causes cardiac arrest with a slow sinusoidal type of mechanism ("sine-wave" pattern) followed by asystole.

Hypocalcemia typically prolongs the QT interval (ST portion), while hypercalcemia shortens it

Digitalis glycosides shortens the QT interval, often with a characteristic "scooping" of the ST–T-wave complex (digitalis effect)

Total electrical alternans (P-QRS-T) with sinus tachycardia is a relatively specific sign of pericardial effusion, usually with cardiac tamponade.

2D echocardiography is the imaging modality of choice for the detection of pericardial effusion---based on modified Bernoulli equation:
Pressure change = 4 x (velocity)^2

Diseases of the aorta, such as aortic dissection, can be readily diagnosed by TEE Defining the source of embolism is a common indication for TEE, as atrial thrombi, patent foramen ovale, and aortic plaques can be detected. Other masses, particularly those in the atria,   presence of vegetations for the diagnosis of infective endocarditis and its complications can be assessed by TEE.

Rubidium-82 is the most commonly used positron emitter-in PET SCAN, pattern of enhanced fluorodeoxyglucose uptake in regions of decreased perfusion (termed glucose/blood flow "mismatch") indicates the presence of ischemic myocardium

MRA is a standard technique for imaging the aorta and large vessels of the chest and abdomen

Limitations of MRI
Relative contraindications include the presence of pacemakers, internal defibrillators, or cerebral aneurysm clips,claustrophobia

renal function deterioration —, that were once common when earlier high-osmolar contrast agents were used. the chance of which may be reduced by adequate prehydration preprocedure administration of N-acetylcysteine , or the use of an isoosmolar contrast agent (iodixanol). Newer low- or iso-osmolar contrast agents also reduce the chance of myocardial depression and other side effects hypotension, nausea, bradycardia.

Imp .

Head-up tilt (HUT) testing is a useful in the evaluation of some patients with syncope

Vaughan-Williams classification— antiarrythmic drugs

definition sinus bradycardia is a rhythm driven by the SA node with a rate of <60 beats/min

AV conduction block has been associated with heritable neuromuscular diseases, eg. the nucleotide repeat disease myotonic dystrophy, the mitochondrial myopathy Kearns-Sayre syndrome

Mobitz type 1 block is characterized by a progressively lengthening PR interval, shortening of the RR interval, and a pause that is less than two times the immediately preceding RR interval on the ECG.

When AV block is 2:1 it may be difficult to distinguish type 1 from type 2 block.

For evaluation of AV block , Vagal maneuvers, carotid sinus massage, exercise, and administration of drugs such as atropine or isoproterenol may be diagnostically and therapeutically important

definition of tachycardia is rhythm that produces a ventricular rate >100 beats/min

Atrial Premature Complexes--- Beta blockers are typical first-line therapy, but they may exacerbate symptoms if AV block occurs with the APC ,IC drugs can be given but not when structural defect is present in heart

Cox surgical Maze procedure is designed to interrupt all macroreentrant circuits— abbelative surgery in AF

Atrioventricular Nodal Reentrant Tachycardia: Treatment---- Vagal stimulation,adenosine first line
Beta blocker-second line

Accelerated Idioventricular Rhythm—three or more complexes at a rate >40 beats/min and <120 beats/min , due to abnormal automaticity.rx-- atropine or by atrial pacing

Fascicular Tachycardia Caused by Digoxin Toxicity

Cheyne-Stokes respiration is common in advanced HF

jugular venous pressure is best appreciated with the patient lying recumbent, with the head tilted at 45°.

Hepatomegaly is an important sign in patients with HF

most useful index of LV function is the EF (stroke volume divided by end-diastolic volume).

Marker of HF.— Both B-type natriuretic peptide (BNP) and N-terminal pro-BNP

Dietary restriction of sodium (2–3 g daily) is recommended in all patients with HF

Drugs blocking the effects of aldosterone =spironolactone or eplerenone

Nesiritide, a vasodilator, is a recombinant form of brain type natriuretic peptide BNP----for HF

Milrinone is a phosphodiesterase III inhibitor that leads to increased cAMP—used in HF

Congenital heart disease (CHD) complicates ~1% of all live births in the general population but occurs in 4% of offspring of women with CHD

Eisenmenger syndrome is applied to predominantly right-to-left shunts because of high-resistance and obstructive pulmonary hypertension.

ASD— common cardiac anomaly that may be first encountered in the adult and occurs more frequently in females

differential cyanosis.—PDA

Bicuspid aortic valves are more common in males than in females

Coarctation of aorta- most common distal to the origin of the left subclavian artery

Indentation of the aorta at the site of coarctation and pre- and poststenotic dilatation (the "3" sign)
Notching of the 3rd to 9th ribs, an important radiographic sign, is due to inferior rib erosion

Valvular pulmonic stenosis is the most common form of isolated RV obstruction

Multiple sites of narrowing of the peripheral pulmonary arteries are a feature of rubella embryopathy

RV hypertrophy.and a normal-sized, boot-shaped heart (coeur en sabot)---TOF

Complete Transposition of the Great Arteries
called dextro- or D-transposition of the great arteries

switch corrections of complete transposition of the great arteries ---the Mustard or Senning operations

mitral valve opening is reduced to <1 cm^2, often referred to as "severe" MS, a LA pressure of ~25 mmHg is required to maintain a normal cardiac output (CO)

Mitral Valve Prolapse
MVP, also called systolic click-murmur syndrome, Barlow's syndrome, floppy-

valve syndrome, and billowing mitral leaflet syndrome

MVP is more common in females autosomal dominant form of inheritance mid- or late (nonejection) systolic click

Laplace relation ($S = Pr/h$, where $S =$ systolic wall stress, $P =$ pressure, $r =$ radius, and $h =$ wall thickness)

paradoxic splitting of S_2 and s4 heard------ aortic stenosis

severe AR is the Austin Flint murmur, a soft, low-pitched, rumbling mid-diastolic murmur

carcinoid syndrome may cause pulmonic stenosis and/or regurgitation

in Peripartum Cardiomyopathy-Cardiac dilatation and CHF may develop during the last trimester of pregnancy or within 6 months of delivery

Trastuzumab (Herceptin), used in the treatment of breast cancer, causes cardiomyopathy in 7% of patients

Arrhythmogenic Right Ventricular Cardiomyopathy—defect in desmosome plakophilin

Tako-Tsubo (Stress) Cardiomyopathy known as apical ballooning syndrome, is characterized by the abrupt onset of severe chest discomfort preceded by a very stressful emotional or physical event. It occurs most commonly in women >50 years and is accompanied by ST-segment elevations and/or deep T-wave
,ballooning of left ventricle offurs

HOCM— The most common are mutations of the cardiac -myosin heavy chain gene on chromosome 14.

hallmark of obstructive HCM is a systolic murmur, which is typically harsh, diamond-shaped

Cardiac Danon Disease—periodic acis Schiff accumulate in myocardium is caused by mutations in an X-linked lysosome-associated membrane protein LAMP2

Hypocalcemia typically prolongs the QT interval (ST portion), while hypercalcemia shortens it

Digitalis glycosides shortens the QT interval, often with a characteristic "scooping" of the ST–T-wave complex (digitalis effect)

Total electrical alternans (P-QRS-T) with sinus tachycardia is a relatively specific sign of pericardial effusion, usually with cardiac tamponade.

2D echocardiography is the imaging modality of choice for the detection of pericardial effusion---based on modified Bernoulli equation:
Pressure change = 4 x (velocity)^2

Diseases of the aorta, such as aortic dissection, can be readily diagnosed by TEE Defining the source of embolism is a common indication for TEE, as atrial thrombi, patent foramen ovale, and aortic plaques can be detected. Other masses, particularly those in the atria,   presence of vegetations for the diagnosis of infective endocarditis and its complications can be assessed by TEE.

Rubidium-82 is the most commonly used positron emitter-in PET SCAN, pattern of enhanced fluorodeoxyglucose uptake in regions of decreased perfusion (termed glucose/blood flow "mismatch") indicates the presence of ischemic myocardium

MRA is a standard technique for imaging the aorta and large vessels of the chest and abdomen

friedrich ataxia (AR) and fabry ds(XR)----
a/w heart l e left ventricular failure

Differentiation of RCM from constrictive
pericarditis---by endomyocardial biopsy

Eosinophilic Endomyocardial Disease
Also called Loeffler's endocarditis and
fibroplastic endocarditis, this occurs in
temperate climates. It is a
hypereosinophilic syndrome

HIV-infected patients have subclinical
cardiac involvement

Lyme ds is tick-borne spirochete . About
10% of patients develop symptomatic
cardiac involvement

Chagas disease, caused by the protozoan Trypanosoma cruzi and transmitted by an insect vector, the reduvid bug, produces an extensive myocarditis

wet beri-beri heart disease is a manifestation of serious thiamine deficiency. It is characterized by cardiac failure secondary to a high cardiac output state

Ewart's sign, and chest roentgenogram may show a "water bottle" in pericardial effusion Echocardiography is the most effective imaging technique

Cardiac tamponade (Beck's triad) are hypotension, soft or absent heart sounds, and jugular venous distention with a prominent x descent but an absent y descent. quantity of fluid necessary to produce this state may be as small as 200 mL

Myxedema may be responsible for chronic pericardial effusion

90% of myxomas are sporadic

NAME syndrome (nevi, atrial myxoma, myxoid neurofibroma, and ephelides)

LAMB syndrome —lentigines, atrial myxoma, and blue nevi

Blunt, nonpenetrating, often innocent-appearing injuries to the chest may trigger ventricular fibrillation even in absence of overt signs of injury. This syndrome, known as commotio cordis

Vitamin B_6, B_{12}, and folate are cofactors in the metabolism of homocysteine—def causes atherosclerosis

carcinoid syndrome have cardiac involvement of the right-sided cardiac structures

Collagen Vascular Diseases—a/w pericarditis

ABCA1, the gene mutated in Tangier disease, characterized by very low HDL levels

Reverse cholesterol transport mediated by ABC transporters

In atherosclerosis--Fatty streak formation begins beneath a morphologically intact endothelium

Rupture of the plaque's fibrous cap allows contact between coagulation factors

more coronary risk in men compared with premenopausal women is well established

hyperhomocysteinemia a/w thrombosis and coronary events

atherosclerosis a/w—homocysteine, Lp(a),
Fibrinogen
CRP,
PAI-1,
myeloperoxidase,
and lipoprotein-associated
phospholipase A_2

Hypertension. interleukin (IL) 1, IL-6, IL-18, resistin, tumor necrosis factor (TNF)=alpha , and C-reactive protein (CRP),   Dyslipidemia, increased Waist Circumference,insulin resistance—a/w metabolic syndrome

Adiponectin is an anti-inflammatory cytokine produced exclusively by adipocytes, Adiponectin is reduced in the metabolic syndrome

fibrate (gemfibrozil or fenofibrate) is the drug of choice to lower fasting triglycerides

drugs that lower triglycerides are statins, nicotinic acid, and high doses of omega-3 fatty acids

NYHA 1-Patients have cardiac disease but without the resulting limitations of physical activity
NYHA 2--cardiac disease resulting in slight limitation of physical activity
NYHA3--cardiac disease resulting in marked limitation of physical activity.
NYHA4--cardiac disease resulting in inability to carry on any physical activity without discomfort.

Aspirin-Chronic administration of 75–325 mg orally per day has been shown to reduce coronary events in asymptomatic adult men

Clopidogrel is an oral agent that blocks ADP receptor–mediated platelet aggregation

Ranolazine, a piperazine derivative, used in chronic angina . drug inhibits the late inward sodium current (I_{Na}).

PCI produces effective relief of angina in >95% of cases

Myocardial perfusion imaging with ^{201}Tl or ^{99m}Tc-sestamib done

fibrinolytic therapy should ideally be initiated within 30 min of presentation in MI

syphilitic aneurysms are located in the ascending aorta or aortic

Tuberculous aneurysms   typically affect the thoracic aorta

mycotic aneurysm is a condition that develops due to bacterial or fungal infections of the aorta, usually at an atherosclerotic plaque. In this case aneurysms are usually saccular, blood culture done

Cystic medial necrosis is the most common cause of ascending aortic aneurysms

Abdominal aortic aneurysms occur more frequently in males than in females

aortic dissection is in the sixth and seventh decades. Men are more affected than women by a ratio of 2:1

Atherosclerotic Occlusive Disease—leriche synd

Giant cell arteritis—affects women more often than men

ankle:brachial index, or ABI) is 1.0 in normal individuals and <1.0 in patients with peripheral arterial disease; a ratio of <0.5 is consistent with severe ischemia

recommends treatment to reduce LDL cholesterol to <100 mg/dL in clinical scenario

most frequently used procedure is the aortobifemoral bypass using knitted Dacron grafts

Fibromuscular Dysplasia
This is a hyperplastic disorder affecting medium-sized and small arteries. It occurs predominantly in females and usually involves renal and carotid arteries

Thromboangiitis Obliterans—— most frequently in men <40 .diagnosis can be confirmed by excisional biopsy

Venous compression may cause thrombosis of the subclavian and axillary veins; this is often associated with effort and referred to as Paget-Schroetter syndrome

Trans-oesophageal echocardiography for—

aortic dissection

Thrombus

Vegetations

Abscess in endocardium

Prosthetic valve abnormality

Left ventricular function

Ischaemia of heart—thallium or technetium scan

Ca^{2+} is stored in the SR by its attachment to a protein, calsequestrin

sarcomere, the structural and functional unit of contraction, lies between two adjacent dark lines, the Z lines

At the center of the sarcomere is a dark band of constant length the A band, which is flanked by two lighter bands, the I bands, which are of variable length.

Titin is a large, flexible, myofibrillar protein that connects myosin to the Z line. Its stretching contributes to the elasticity of the heart.

calcium ion activates the myosin ATPase

Ca^{2+} becomes attached to troponin C, which results in a conformational change in the regulatory protein tropomyosin;

which exposes the actin cross-bridge interaction sites

Laplace's law says that the tension of myocardial fiber is a function of the product of the intracavitary ventricular pressure and ventricular radius divided by the wall thickness. so at particular level of aortic pressure, afterload on a dilated left ventricle is higher than that on a non dilated ventricle.

bisferiens pulse, which has two systolic peaks is feature of aortic regurgitation

Hypertrophic Obstructive Cardiomyopathy (HOCM)

is an autosomal dominant

disorder of muscle tissue caused by defects in the genes encoding contractile proteins.

The estimated

prevalence is 1 in 500.

Septal hypertrophy causes left ventricular outflow obstruction. It is an

important cause of sudden death in apparently healthy individuals.

Hypertrophic obstructive cardiomyopathy (HOCM) is a common cause of sudden cardiac death than arrhythmogenic right ventricular dysplasia (ARVD) 2nd most common

Often asymptomatic

Dyspnea, angina, syncope

Sudden death (most commonly due to ventricular arrhythmias), arrhythmias, heart failure

Jerky pulse,

large 'a' waves

, double apex beat

Ejection systolic murmur: _ with valsalva manoeuvre and _ on squatting

a/w

Friedreich's ataxia

Wolff-Parkinson White syndrome

Left ventricular hypertrophy (LVH)

Atrial enlargement (abnormal P morphology)

Progressive T wave inversion

ST-T abnormalities

Deep Q waves

Axis deviation

Prolonged PR or sinus bradycardia

BBB (bundle brach block)

No P waves and irregular narrow QRS complexes This is hallmark of atrial fibrillation

---

www.ingramcontent.com/pod-product-compliance
Lightning Source LLC
Chambersburg PA
CBHW070825180526
45168CB00002B/743